Copyright © 2023 by N

All rights reserved. No part of this publication may be reproduced, distributed, or transmitted in any form or by any means, including photocopying, recording, or other electronic or mechanical methods, without the prior written permission of the publisher, except in the case of brief quotations embodied in critical reviews and certain other noncommercial uses permitted by copyright law.

Table of Contents

INDIGESTION 4

INDIGESTION RECIPES 5

   1. Frittata with Asparagus, Leek & Ricotta 5

   2. 3-Ingredient Baked Feta & Cherry Tomato Egg Muffins 7

   3. 3-Ingredient Overnight Berry Muesli 9

   4. Mixed-Berry Breakfast Smoothie 10

   5. Muffin-Tin Spinach & Mushroom Mini Quiches 11

   6. Spinach & Egg Scramble with Raspberries 13

   7. Lemon-Blueberry Yogurt Toast 15

   8. Muffin-Tin Omelets with Feta & Peppers 17

   9. Egg Sandwiches with Rosemary, Tomato & Feta 19

   10. Spinach, Mushroom & Egg Casserole 21

   11. Peanut Butter-Banana English Muffin 23

   12. Zucchini, Corn & Egg Casserole 24

   13. Baked Eggs in Tomato Sauce with Kale 26

   14. Muffin-Tin Omelets with Bell Pepper, Black Beans & Jack Cheese 28

   15. White Bean & Avocado Toast 30

   16. Baked Blueberry & Banana-Nut Oatmeal Cups 31

   17. Chocolate-Banana Protein Smoothie 33

   18. "Egg in a Hole" Peppers with Avocado Salsa 34

   19. Spinach & Egg Scramble with Raspberries 36

   20. Sriracha, Egg & Avocado Overnight Oats 38

   21. Spiralized Zucchini Nest Eggs 39

22. Muffin-Tin Omelets with Veggie Sausage & Sun-Dried Tomatoes 41

23. Turkey Burgers with Spinach, Feta & Tzatziki 43

24. Instant-Pot Chicken Burrito Bowl 45

25. Sheet-Pan Chicken Cutlets with Brussels Sprouts & Sweet Potatoes 48

26. Garlicky Pasta with Grilled Shrimp & Asparagus 50

27. Vegetarian Protein Bowl 52

28. Cilantro-Lime Shrimp Bowl 55

29. Garlic-Anchovy Pasta with Broccolini 58

30. Cheesy Ground Beef & Broccoli Casserole 60

INDIGESTION

Indigestion — also called dyspepsia or an upset stomach — is discomfort in your upper abdomen. Indigestion describes certain symptoms, such as abdominal pain and a feeling of fullness soon after you start eating, rather than a specific disease. Indigestion can also be a symptom of various digestive diseases.

INDIGESTION RECIPES

1. Frittata with Asparagus, Leek & Ricotta

Prep Time: 20 mins

Total Time: 20 mins

Servings: 4

Ingredients

- 8 large eggs
- ¼ cup crème fraîche
- ½ teaspoon salt
- ¼ teaspoon ground pepper
- 2 tablespoons extra-virgin olive oil
- 3 cups thinly sliced leeks (about 2 medium), rinsed well and patted dry
- 1 pound asparagus, trimmed and cut into 1-inch pieces
- ¼ cup part-skim ricotta
- 2 tablespoons pesto
- ¼ cup fresh basil

Directions

1. Position rack in upper third of oven; preheat broiler.
2. Whisk eggs, crème fraîche, salt and pepper in a medium bowl; set near the stove. Heat oil in a large cast-iron skillet over medium-high heat. Add leeks and asparagus and cook, stirring frequently, until soft, 5 to 6 minutes.
3. Pour the egg mixture over the vegetables and cook, lifting the edges so uncooked egg can flow underneath, until nearly set, about 2 minutes. Dollop ricotta and pesto on top and place the pan under the broiler until the eggs are slightly browned, 1 1/2 to 2 minutes. Let stand for 3 minutes.
4. Run a spatula around the edge of the frittata, then underneath, until you can slide or lift it out onto a cutting board or serving plate. Top with basil.

2. 3-Ingredient Baked Feta & Cherry Tomato Egg Muffins

Prep Time: 10 mins

Total Time: 40 mins

Servings: 4

Ingredients

- 1 ½ cups cherry tomatoes, halved
- 2 ounces feta cheese, cubed
- 6 large eggs
- ¼ teaspoon salt
- Ground pepper to taste
- Thinly sliced fresh basil for garnish

Directions

1. Preheat oven to 325°F. Coat 8 muffin-tin cups with cooking spray or use silicone muffin-tin liners.
2. Divide tomatoes and feta among the prepared cups. Whisk eggs, salt and pepper to taste in a medium bowl. Pour the eggs over the tomatoes and feta in the muffin cups. Top with basil, if desired.
3. Bake until the eggs are set, 20 to 25 minutes. Let cool in the pan for 5 minutes before serving. If not

serving immediately, transfer to a wire rack to cool completely before refrigerating for up to 4 days or freezing for up to 3 months.

3. 3-Ingredient Overnight Berry Muesli

Prep Time: 5 mins

Total Time: 8 hrs

Servings: 4

Ingredients

- 1 cup muesli
- 2 cups plain kefir
- 2 cups frozen mixed berries

Directions

1. Spoon ¼ cup muesli into each of 4 jars or containers. Top each with ½ cup kefir and ½ cup frozen berries; mix well to combine. Cover and refrigerate overnight, or for up to 4 days. Stir well before serving.

4. Mixed-Berry Breakfast Smoothie

Prep Time: 5 mins

Total Time: 5 mins

Servings: 1

Ingredients

- 1 cup frozen mixed berries
- ¾ cup water
- ½ cup low-fat plain Greek yogurt
- 1 banana
- ¼ avocado
- 2 tablespoons chopped walnuts

Directions

1. Combine berries, water, yogurt, banana, avocado and walnuts in a blender. Blend on high speed until smooth. If necessary, add more water to reach desired consistency.

5. Muffin-Tin Spinach & Mushroom Mini Quiches

Prep Time: 35 mins

Total Time: 1 hr 5 mins

Servings: 6

Ingredients

- 2 tablespoons extra-virgin olive oil
- 8 ounces fresh mixed wild mushrooms
- 1 cup thinly sliced yellow onion
- 1 tablespoon minced garlic
- 2 teaspoons minced fresh thyme
- 1 (5 ounce) package fresh spinach, coarsely chopped
- 8 large eggs
- ⅔ cup whole milk
- 2 teaspoons Dijon mustard
- ½ teaspoon salt
- ½ teaspoon ground pepper
- ¾ cup shredded Gruyère cheese

Directions

1. Preheat oven to 325 degrees F. Heat oil in a large nonstick skillet over medium-high heat. Add mushrooms in an even layer; cook, undisturbed, until browned on the bottom, about 4 minutes. Stir and continue to cook, stirring occasionally, until browned all over, about 5 minutes. Add onion; cook, stirring occasionally, until beginning to soften, about 4 minutes. Stir in garlic and thyme; cook, stirring, until fragrant, about 2 minutes. Add spinach; cook, stirring constantly, until just wilted, about 2 minutes. Remove from heat.
2. Whisk eggs, milk, Dijon, salt and pepper in a large bowl. Stir in cheese and the mushroom mixture. Coat a standard 12-cup muffin tin with cooking spray. Divide the mixture among the prepared muffin cups. Bake, uncovered, until puffed and set, about 30 minutes. Remove from the pan and serve immediately.

6. Spinach & Egg Scramble with Raspberries

Prep Time: 10 mins

Total Time: 10 mins

Servings: 1

Ingredients

- 1 teaspoon canola oil
- 1 ½ cups baby spinach (1 1/2 ounces)
- 2 large eggs, lightly beaten
- Pinch of kosher salt
- Pinch of ground pepper
- 1 slice whole-grain bread, toasted
- ½ cup fresh raspberries

Directions

1. Heat oil in a small nonstick skillet over medium-high heat. Add spinach and cook until wilted, stirring often, 1 to 2 minutes. Transfer the spinach to a plate. Wipe the pan clean, place over medium heat and add eggs. Cook, stirring once or twice to ensure even cooking, until just set, 1 to 2 minutes.

Stir in the spinach, salt and pepper. Serve the scramble with toast and raspberries.

7. Lemon-Blueberry Yogurt Toast

Prep Time: 5 mins

Total Time: 20 mins

Servings: 2

Ingredients

- 1 large egg
- 3 tablespoons plain whole-milk strained yogurt
- 1 tablespoon pure maple syrup
- 1 teaspoon lemon zest
- 1 teaspoon lemon juice
- Pinch of salt
- 2 slices whole-wheat bread, 1/2 inch thick
- ¼ cup fresh blueberries

Directions

1. Preheat oven to 375°F. Line a baking sheet with parchment paper. Whisk together egg, yogurt, maple syrup, lemon zest, lemon juice and salt in a small bowl.
2. Place bread on the prepared baking sheet. Using your fingers or the back of a spoon, press down on

the center of each slice, making a large indentation and leaving a 1/2-inch border between the indentation and the crust. Spoon the yogurt mixture into the indentation and spread evenly. Top with blueberries. Bake until the yogurt mixture is set and the blueberries have started to burst, 8 to 10 minutes. Let cool slightly, about 5 minutes.

8. Muffin-Tin Omelets with Feta & Peppers

Prep Time: 25 mins

Total Time: 50 mins

Servings: 6

Ingredients

- 2 tablespoons extra-virgin olive oil
- ¾ cup diced onion
- ¼ teaspoon salt, divided
- 1 medium red bell pepper, diced
- 1 tablespoon finely chopped fresh oregano
- 8 large eggs
- ¾ cup crumbled feta cheese
- ½ cup low-fat milk
- ½ teaspoon ground pepper
- 2 cups chopped fresh spinach
- ¼ cup sliced Kalamata olives

Directions

1. Preheat oven to 325 degrees F. Liberally coat a 12-cup muffin tin with cooking spray.

2. Heat oil in a large skillet over medium heat. Add onion and 1/8 teaspoon salt; cook, stirring, until starting to soften, about 3 minutes. Add bell pepper and oregano; cook, stirring, until the vegetables are tender and starting to brown, 4 to 5 minutes more. Remove from heat and let cool for 5 minutes.
3. Whisk eggs, feta, milk, pepper and the remaining 1/8 teaspoon salt in a large bowl. Stir in spinach, olives and the vegetable mixture. Divide among the prepared muffin cups.
4. Bake until firm to the touch, about 25 minutes. Let stand for 5 minutes before removing from the tin.

9. Egg Sandwiches with Rosemary, Tomato & Feta

Prep Time: 5 mins

Total Time: 20 mins

Servings: 4

Ingredients

- 4 multigrain sandwich thins
- 4 teaspoons olive oil
- 1 tablespoon snipped fresh rosemary or 1/2 teaspoon dried rosemary, crushed
- 4 eggs
- 2 cups fresh baby spinach leaves
- 1 medium tomato, cut into 8 thin slices
- 4 tablespoons reduced-fat feta cheese
- ⅛ teaspoon kosher salt

Directions

1. Preheat oven to 375 degrees F. Split sandwich thins; brush cut sides with 2 teaspoons of the olive oil. Place on rimmed baking sheet; toast in oven about 5 minutes or until edges are light brown and crisp.

2. Meanwhile, in a large skillet heat the remaining 2 teaspoons olive oil and the rosemary over medium-high heat. Break eggs, one at a time, into skillet. Cook about 1 minute or until whites are set but yolks are still runny. Break yolks with spatula. Flip eggs; cook on other side until done. Remove from heat.
3. Place the bottom halves of the toasted sandwich thins on four serving plates. Divide spinach among sandwich thins on plates. Top each with two of the tomato slices, an egg and 1 tablespoon of the feta cheese. Sprinkle with the salt and pepper. Top with the remaining sandwich thin halves.

10. Spinach, Mushroom & Egg Casserole

Prep Time: 25 mins

Total Time: 1 hr 5 mins

Servings: 10

Ingredients

- 2 tablespoons extra-virgin olive oil
- 1 pound cremini mushrooms, trimmed and sliced
- 5 medium cloves garlic, finely chopped
- 2 teaspoons dry mustard
- 1 teaspoon onion powder
- 1 teaspoon salt
- 5 ounces baby spinach
- 12 large eggs
- ¾ cup half-and-half
- 1 ½ cups shredded Gruyère cheese, preferably cave-aged, divided
- 2 teaspoons fresh thyme leaves

Directions

1. Preheat oven to 375°F. Coat a 9-by-13-inch baking dish with cooking spray. Heat oil in a large skillet

over medium-high heat. Add mushrooms in an even layer; cook, undisturbed, until starting to brown, 5 to 6 minutes. Stir and continue to cook, undisturbed, until golden brown on the bottom, about 3 minutes. Stir and continue to cook, stirring occasionally, until the mushrooms are browned all over and the liquid has evaporated, about 3 minutes. Add garlic, dry mustard, onion powder and salt; cook, stirring constantly, until fragrant, about 1 minute. Add spinach and cook, stirring constantly, until the spinach wilts, 1 to 2 minutes. Set aside to cool slightly, about 10 minutes.

2. Crack eggs into a large bowl and whisk until completely smooth. Add half-and-half and whisk until combined. Reserve 1/2 cup of the vegetable mixture; scatter the remaining mixture in the prepared baking dish. Sprinkle evenly with 3/4 cup Gruyère. Pour the egg mixture over the top. Sprinkle evenly with the remaining 3/4 cup Gruyère and the reserved 1/2 cup vegetable mixture. Bake until puffed, golden brown and just set, 30 to 35 minutes. Let cool slightly, about 10 minutes. Sprinkle with thyme before serving.

11. Peanut Butter-Banana English Muffin

Prep Time: 5 mins

Total Time: 5 mins

Servings: 1

Ingredients

- 1 whole-wheat English muffin, toasted
- 1 tablespoon peanut butter
- ½ banana, sliced
- Pinch of ground cinnamon

Directions

1. Top English muffin with peanut butter, banana and cinnamon.

12. Zucchini, Corn & Egg Casserole

Total Time: 1 hr 15 mins

Servings: 8

Ingredients

- 5 cups shredded zucchini and/or summer squash (about 3 medium)
- 2 tablespoons butter
- 1 cup finely chopped onion
- Pinch of salt, plus 1/4 teaspoon, divided
- 1 ½ cups corn kernels, fresh or frozen
- 1 ¼ cups no-salt-added cottage cheese
- 1 cup crumbled feta cheese
- ½ cup chopped red bell pepper
- ¼ cup chopped fresh dill
- 2 tablespoons all-purpose flour
- 1 teaspoon baking powder
- ¼ teaspoon ground pepper
- 10 large eggs, lightly beaten

Directions

1. Preheat oven to 350 degrees F. Coat a 9-by-13-inch baking dish (or similar-size 3-quart baking dish) with cooking spray.
2. Place squash on a clean kitchen towel, gather up the edges and squeeze out excess moisture.
3. Heat butter in a large skillet over medium heat. Add onion and cook, stirring occasionally, until golden brown, 5 to 8 minutes. Add the squash and a pinch of salt; cook until very soft and dry; about 4 minutes more.
4. Transfer the squash mixture to a large bowl. Add corn, cottage cheese, feta, bell pepper, dill, flour, baking powder, pepper and the remaining 1/4 teaspoon salt and stir until well combined. Stir in eggs. Pour the mixture into the prepared baking dish.
5. Bake the casserole until the center is set and the edges are lightly browned, about 40 minutes. Let stand 10 minutes before serving.

13. Baked Eggs in Tomato Sauce with Kale

Prep Time: 10 mins

Total Time: 30 mins

Servings: 4

Ingredients

- 1 tablespoon extra-virgin olive oil
- 3 10-ounce packages frozen chopped kale, thawed, drained and squeezed dry (9 cups)
- ½ teaspoon salt, divided
- ¼ teaspoon ground pepper, divided
- 1 25-ounce jar low-sodium marinara sauce or 3 cups canned low-sodium tomato sauce
- 8 large eggs

Directions

1. Preheat oven to 350 degrees F.
2. Heat oil in a 10-inch cast-iron skillet or nonstick ovenproof skillet over medium heat. Add kale, season with 1/4 teaspoon salt and 1/8 teaspoon pepper, and sauté for 2 minutes. Stir in marinara (or tomato) sauce and bring to a simmer.

3. Make 8 wells in the sauce with the back of a spoon and carefully crack an egg into each well. Season the eggs with the remaining 1/4 teaspoon salt and 1/8 teaspoon pepper.
4. Transfer the pan to the oven and bake until the egg whites are set and the yolks are still soft, about 20 minutes.

14. Muffin-Tin Omelets with Bell Pepper, Black Beans & Jack Cheese

Prep Time: 20 mins

Total Time: 45 mins

Servings: 6

Ingredients

- 8 large eggs
- ½ cup reduced-fat milk
- ¼ teaspoon salt
- ¼ teaspoon ground pepper
- ¾ cup chopped red bell pepper
- ¾ cup black beans, rinsed
- 6 tablespoons shredded Monterey Jack cheese
- ¼ cup salsa

Directions

1. Preheat oven to 325 degrees F.
2. Whisk eggs, milk, salt and pepper in a large bowl.
3. Liberally coat a 12-cup muffin pan with cooking spray (or use silicone muffin cups). Divide bell pepper, black beans, cheese and salsa among the muffin cups. Top with the egg mixture. Bake until

set and lightly brown, 20 to 25 minutes. Let stand for 5 minutes before removing from the pan.

15. White Bean & Avocado Toast

Prep Time: 5 mins

Total Time: 5 mins

Servings: 1

Ingredients

- 1 slice whole-wheat bread, toasted
- ¼ avocado, mashed
- ½ cup canned white beans, rinsed and drained
- Kosher salt to taste
- Ground pepper to taste
- 1 pinch Crushed red pepper

Directions

1. Top toast with mashed avocado and white beans. Season with a pinch each of salt, pepper and crushed red pepper.

16. Baked Blueberry & Banana-Nut Oatmeal Cups

Prep Time: 15 mins

Total Time: 50 mins

Servings: 12

Ingredients

- 3 cups oats
- 1 ½ cups low-fat milk
- 2 ripe bananas, mashed (about 3/4 cup)
- ⅓ cup packed brown sugar
- 2 large eggs, lightly beaten
- 1 teaspoon baking powder
- 1 teaspoon ground cinnamon
- 1 teaspoon vanilla extract
- ½ teaspoon salt
- 1 cup fresh blueberries
- ½ cup chopped toasted pecans

Directions

1. Preheat oven to 375°F. Coat a muffin tin with cooking spray.

2. Combine oats, milk, bananas, brown sugar, eggs, baking powder, cinnamon, vanilla and salt in a large bowl. Fold in blueberries and pecans. Divide the mixture between the muffin cups (about 1/3 cup each). Bake until a toothpick inserted into the center comes out clean, about 25 minutes. Cool in the pan for 10 minutes, then turn out onto a wire rack. Serve warm or at room temperature.

17. Chocolate-Banana Protein Smoothie

Prep Time: 5 mins

Total Time: 5 mins

Servings: 1

Ingredients

- 1 banana, frozen
- ½ cup cooked red lentils
- ½ cup nonfat milk
- 2 teaspoons unsweetened cocoa powder
- 1 teaspoon pure maple syrup

Directions

1. Combine banana, lentils, milk, cocoa and syrup in a blender. Puree until smooth.

18. "Egg in a Hole" Peppers with Avocado Salsa

Prep Time: 35 mins

Total Time: 35 mins

Servings: 4

Ingredients

- 2 bell peppers, any color
- 1 avocado, diced
- ½ cup diced red onion
- 1 jalapeño pepper, minced
- ½ cup chopped fresh cilantro, plus more for garnish
- 2 tomatoes, seeded and diced
- Juice of 1 lime
- ¾ teaspoon salt, divided
- 2 teaspoons olive oil, divided
- 8 large eggs
- ¼ teaspoon ground pepper, divided

Directions

1. Slice tops and bottoms off bell peppers and finely dice. Remove and discard seeds and membranes. Slice each pepper into four 1/2-inch-thick rings.
2. Combine the diced pepper with avocado, onion, jalapeño, cilantro, tomatoes, lime juice, and 1/2 teaspoon salt in a medium bowl.
3. Heat 1 teaspoon oil in a large nonstick skillet over medium heat. Add 4 bell pepper rings, then crack 1 egg into the middle of each ring. Season with 1/8 teaspoon each salt and pepper. Cook until the whites are mostly set but the yolks are still runny, 2 to 3 minutes. Gently flip and cook 1 minute more for runny yolks, 1 1/2 to 2 minutes more for firmer yolks. Transfer to serving plates and repeat with the remaining pepper rings and eggs.
4. Serve with the avocado salsa and garnish with additional cilantro, if desired.

19. Spinach & Egg Scramble with Raspberries

Prep Time: 10 mins

Total Time: 10 mins

Servings: 1

Ingredients

- 1 teaspoon canola oil
- 1 ½ cups baby spinach (1 1/2 ounces)
- 2 large eggs, lightly beaten
- Pinch of kosher salt
- Pinch of ground pepper
- 1 slice whole-grain bread, toasted
- ½ cup fresh raspberries

Directions

1. Heat oil in a small nonstick skillet over medium-high heat. Add spinach and cook until wilted, stirring often, 1 to 2 minutes. Transfer the spinach to a plate. Wipe the pan clean, place over medium heat and add eggs. Cook, stirring once or twice to ensure even cooking, until just set, 1 to 2 minutes.

Stir in the spinach, salt and pepper. Serve the scramble with toast and raspberries

20. Sriracha, Egg & Avocado Overnight Oats

Prep Time: 15 mins

Total Time: 8 hrs

Servings: 1

Ingredients

- ½ cup rolled oats
- ¾ cup water
- 1 tablespoon onion
- ¼ avocado, sliced
- 2 cherry tomatoes, chopped
- 1 large egg, fried
- 1 teaspoon Sriracha

Directions

1. Combine oats and water in a small bowl or jar. Cover and refrigerate overnight.
2. Stir in onion and microwave in 30-second intervals, stirring occasionally, until heated through. Arrange in a bowl with avocado and tomatoes. Top with the egg and Sriracha.

21. Spiralized Zucchini Nest Eggs

Prep Time: 25 mins

Total Time: 40 mins

Servings: 4

Ingredients

- 2 medium zucchini (1 pound), spiralized
- 1 tablespoon extra-virgin olive oil
- ¼ teaspoon ground pepper, divided
- ¼ teaspoon salt
- ¼ teaspoon garlic powder
- ½ cup part-skim ricotta
- ¼ cup chopped fresh basil
- 2 tablespoons grated Parmesan cheese
- 4 medium eggs

Directions

1. Preheat oven to 400 degrees F. Coat a large rimmed baking sheet with cooking spray.
2. Toss zucchini with oil, 1/8 teaspoon pepper, salt and garlic powder until evenly coated. Using 1 cup

zucchini each, create 4 nests on the prepared pan. Bake for 5 minutes.

3. Meanwhile, stir ricotta, basil, Parmesan and the remaining 1/8 teaspoon pepper together in a small bowl. Spread 2 tablespoons of the mixture in the center of each nest, creating an indentation. Crack an egg into each indentation. (It's OK if some of the egg spills out.) Bake until desired doneness, 12 to 15 minutes for medium set or 14 to 18 minutes for hard set.

22. Muffin-Tin Omelets with Veggie Sausage & Sun-Dried Tomatoes

Prep Time: 20 mins

Total Time: 45 mins

Servings: 6

Ingredients

- 8 large eggs
- ½ cup reduced-fat milk
- ¼ teaspoon salt
- ¼ teaspoon ground pepper
- ¾ cup chopped roasted red peppers
- ¾ cup crumbled cooked veggie sausage
- 6 tablespoons mozzarella cheese
- ¼ cup chopped sun-dried tomatoes

Directions

1. Preheat oven to 325 degrees F.
2. Whisk eggs, milk, salt and pepper in a large bowl.
3. Liberally coat a 12-cup muffin pan with cooking spray (or use silicone muffin cups). Divide roasted red peppers, veggie sausage, mozzarella and sun-dried tomatoes among the muffin cups. Top with

the egg mixture. Bake until set and lightly brown, 20 to 25 minutes. Let stand for 5 minutes before removing from the pan.

23. Turkey Burgers with Spinach, Feta & Tzatziki

Prep Time: 30 mins

Total Time: 30 mins

Servings: 4

Ingredients

- 1 cup frozen chopped spinach, thawed
- 1 pound 93% lean ground turkey
- ½ cup crumbled feta cheese
- ½ teaspoon garlic powder
- ½ teaspoon dried oregano
- ¼ teaspoon salt
- ¼ teaspoon ground pepper
- 4 small hamburger buns, preferably whole-wheat, split
- 4 tablespoons tzatziki
- 12 slices cucumber
- 8 thick rings red onion (about 1/4-inch)

Directions

1. Preheat grill to medium-high. Squeeze excess moisture from spinach. Combine the spinach with

turkey, feta, garlic powder, oregano, salt and pepper in a medium bowl; mix well. Form into four 4-inch patties. Oil the grill rack. Grill the patties until cooked through and no longer pink in the center, 4 to 6 minutes per side. (An instant-read thermometer inserted in the center should register 165°F.) Assemble the burgers on the buns, topping each with 1 tablespoon tzatziki, 3 cucumber slices and 2 onion rings.

24. Instant-Pot Chicken Burrito Bowl

Prep Time: 25 mins

Total Time: 40 mins

Servings: 4

Ingredients

- 2 tablespoons extra-virgin olive oil, divided
- 1 pound boneless, skinless chicken breasts
- 1 cup chopped yellow onion
- 1 tablespoon chopped garlic
- 1 teaspoon ground cumin
- 1 teaspoon ground coriander
- 1 teaspoon dried oregano
- ½ teaspoon salt
- ½ teaspoon ground pepper
- 1 (14.5 ounce) can fire roasted diced tomatoes
- 2 cups hot cooked brown rice
- 1 cup rinsed canned no-salt-added black beans, warmed
- 1 cup frozen corn, warmed
- 1 avocado, chopped
- ¼ cup chopped fresh cilantro

- ½ cup crumbled queso fresco
- Lime wedges for serving

Directions

1. Select Sauté setting on a programmable pressure multicooker (such as Instant Pot; times, instructions and settings may vary according to cooker brand or model). Select High temperature setting, add 1 tablespoon oil to the cooker and allow to preheat for 1 to 2 minutes. Add chicken; cook, turning once, until golden brown on both sides, 3 to 4 minutes per side. Transfer the chicken to a plate.
2. Add the remaining 1 tablespoon oil to the cooker and stir in onion. Cook, stirring often, until translucent, 2 to 5 minutes. Stir in garlic, cumin, coriander, oregano, salt and pepper; cook, stirring constantly, until aromatic, about 30 seconds. Add tomatoes and stir to combine. Return the chicken to the cooker. Press Cancel.
3. Cover the cooker and lock the lid in place. Turn the steam release handle to Sealing position. Select Manual/Pressure Cook setting. Select High

pressure for 7 minutes. (It will take 6 to 8 minutes for the cooker to come up to pressure before cooking begins.)

4. When cooking is complete, carefully turn the steam release handle to Venting position and let the steam fully escape (the float valve will drop; this will take 2 to 3 minutes). Check that an instant-read thermometer inserted in the thickest portion of the chicken registers at least 165°F.

5. Shred the chicken using two forks (this can be done in the cooker for ease). Divide rice evenly among 4 bowls. Top evenly with chicken, black beans, corn, avocado, cilantro and queso fresco. Serve with lime wedges, if desired.

25. Sheet-Pan Chicken Cutlets with Brussels Sprouts & Sweet Potatoes

Prep Time: 15 mins

Total Time: 40 mins

Servings: 4

Ingredients

- 1 pound sweet potatoes, scrubbed and cut into 1/2-inch wedges
- 2 tablespoons extra-virgin olive oil, divided
- ¾ teaspoon salt, divided
- ¾ teaspoon ground pepper, divided
- 4 cups Brussels sprouts, trimmed and halved or quartered if large
- 1 ¼ pounds chicken cutlets
- 1 teaspoon ground fennel
- 3 tablespoons crumbled cooked bacon

Directions

1. Position rack in bottom third of oven; preheat to 425°F.
2. Toss sweet potatoes with 1 tablespoon oil and 1/4 teaspoon each salt and pepper in a large bowl.

Spread evenly on a large rimmed baking sheet. Roast for 15 minutes.
3. Toss Brussels sprouts with the remaining 1 tablespoon oil and 1/4 teaspoon each salt and pepper in the bowl. Stir into the sweet potatoes on the baking sheet.
4. Sprinkle chicken with fennel and the remaining 1/4 teaspoon each salt and pepper. Place on top of the vegetables. Roast until the chicken is cooked through and the vegetables are tender, 15 to 20 minutes more.
5. Transfer the chicken to a serving platter. Stir bacon into the vegetables and serve with the chicken.

26. Garlicky Pasta with Grilled Shrimp & Asparagus

Prep Time: 35 mins

Total Time: 35 mins

Servings: 6

Ingredients

- 1 pound penne, preferably whole-wheat
- 2 tablespoons unsalted butter
- 3 cloves garlic, minced
- 1 ½ cups low-sodium chicken broth
- ½ cup heavy cream
- 2 tablespoons lemon juice, or more to taste
- ½ teaspoon salt, divided
- ½ teaspoon ground pepper, divided
- ⅓ cup grated Romano cheese
- 1 pound large shrimp (21-30 count), peeled and deveined
- 12 ounces asparagus, trimmed

Directions

1. Preheat grill to medium.

2. Bring a large saucepan of water to a boil. Cook penne according to package directions. Drain.
3. Meanwhile, heat butter in a large skillet over medium heat. Add garlic and cook, stirring, for 1 minute. Add broth, cream, lemon juice and 1/4 teaspoon each salt and pepper; bring to a simmer. Reduce heat to maintain a simmer and cook, stirring occasionally, until slightly thickened, about 10 minutes. Stir in cheese and the penne.
4. Meanwhile, lightly coat shrimp and asparagus with cooking spray and sprinkle with the remaining 1/4 teaspoon each salt and pepper. Grill, turning once, until the shrimp are opaque and the asparagus is tender, 4 to 6 minutes.
5. When cool enough to handle, chop asparagus and stir into the pasta. Serve topped with the grilled shrimp.

27. Vegetarian Protein Bowl

Prep Time: 30 mins

Total Time: 1 hr

Servings: 4

Ingredients

- 8 cups water
- 1 ¼ cups farro
- 1 (15 ounce) can no-salt-added cannellini beans, rinsed
- 4 cups cauliflower florets
- 1 (1 pound) sweet potato, peeled and cut into 1-inch cubes
- 2 tablespoons extra-virgin olive oil plus 1/4 cup, divided
- 2 teaspoons lemon-pepper seasoning, divided
- ¾ teaspoon salt, divided
- 1 (6-ounce) bunch fresh broccolini, cut into 2-inch pieces
- ½ cup chopped fresh flat-leaf parsley
- ¼ cup chopped fresh cilantro
- 1 tablespoon red-wine vinegar

- 1 large clove garlic, grated
- ½ teaspoon crushed red pepper
- ¼ cup chopped Castelvetrano olives

Directions

1. Preheat oven to 425°F. Line a large rimmed baking sheet with parchment paper. Bring water to a boil in a large saucepan over medium-high heat; stir in farro. Return to a boil; reduce heat to medium and cook at a low boil, undisturbed, until the grains have expanded but are still al dente, about 30 minutes, stirring in cannellini beans during the last 5 minutes of cooking. Remove from heat and drain. Cover to keep warm.

2. Meanwhile, place cauliflower florets and sweet potato on the prepared baking sheet. Drizzle with 1 1/2 tablespoons oil and sprinkle with 1 1/2 teaspoons lemon-pepper and 1/4 teaspoon salt; toss well to coat and spread evenly on the pan. Combine broccolini, 1/2 tablespoon oil and the remaining 1/2 teaspoon lemon-pepper in a medium bowl and toss to coat; set aside. Roast the sweet potato and cauliflower until almost tender,

about 20 minutes. Remove from oven and push the sweet potatoes and cauliflower to one side. Add the broccolini to other side of the pan; roast until the vegetables are tender and lightly charred, about 10 minutes.

3. Meanwhile, stir parsley, cilantro, vinegar, garlic, crushed red pepper, olives and the remaining 1/4 cup oil and 1/2 teaspoon salt together in a small bowl to make chimichurri. Stir 1/4 cup of the chimichurri into the farro mixture.

4. Divide the farro mixture among 4 bowls and top evenly with roasted vegetables; drizzle with the remaining 1/4 cup chimichurri.

28. Cilantro-Lime Shrimp Bowl

Prep Time: 30 mins

Total Time: 30 mins

Servings: 4

Ingredients

- 1 (15 ounce) can no-salt-added black beans, rinsed
- 1 cup fresh corn kernels (from 2 ears) or 1 cup thawed frozen corn
- ¾ teaspoon salt, divided
- ½ teaspoon ground pepper, divided
- 1 (4-ounce) can Hatch chiles, undrained
- ¼ cup plain whole-milk strained yogurt
- 1 serrano chile, stemmed
- 3 tablespoons avocado oil, divided
- 1 teaspoon grated lime zest
- 4 tablespoons lime juice, divided
- 2 tablespoons finely chopped garlic, divided
- 1 pound large raw shrimp, peeled and deveined
- ½ cup chopped fresh cilantro, plus more for garnish
- 2 cups hot cooked brown rice

- 1 avocado, sliced
- Lime wedges for serving

Directions

1. Combine black beans, corn and 1/4 teaspoon each salt and pepper in a medium bowl. Set aside.
2. Combine Hatch chiles, yogurt, serrano, 1 tablespoon oil, 1 tablespoon lime juice, 1/2 tablespoon garlic and 1/4 teaspoon salt in a blender; process until smooth, about 1 minute. Set the yogurt sauce aside.
3. Toss shrimp with the remaining 1 1/2 tablespoons garlic and 1/4 teaspoon each salt and pepper. Heat the remaining 2 tablespoons oil in a large nonstick skillet over medium-high heat. Add the shrimp in a single layer and cook, undisturbed, for 4 minutes. Add lime zest, cilantro and the remaining 3 tablespoons lime juice; stir to combine. Cook, stirring often, until the shrimp are opaque, 2 to 3 minutes.
4. Divide rice, shrimp, black bean mixture and avocado evenly among 4 bowls and drizzle with

yogurt sauce. Garnish with additional cilantro and serve with lime wedges, if desired.

29. Garlic-Anchovy Pasta with Broccolini

Prep Time: 25 mins

Total Time: 25 mins

Servings: 4

Ingredients

- 2 tablespoons extra-virgin olive oil
- 6 anchovy fillets
- 4 cloves garlic, thinly sliced
- Pinch of crushed red pepper
- 1 (5 ounce) package baby spinach
- 8 ounces whole-wheat angel hair pasta
- 2 bunches broccolini or 1 bunch broccoli rabe, trimmed and coarsely chopped
- ¼ cup chopped fresh parsley
- ¼ teaspoon salt
- ½ cup chopped almonds, toasted
- 4 ounces goat cheese, crumbled
- Grated lemon zest for garnish

Directions

1. Put a large pot of water on to boil.

2. Meanwhile, heat oil in a large skillet over medium heat. Add anchovies, garlic and crushed red pepper; cook, pressing the anchovies with the back of a wooden spoon to break them up, until fragrant, about 2 minutes. Add spinach in 2 batches and cook, stirring occasionally, until just wilted, about 1 minute. Remove from heat and cover to keep warm.
3. Add pasta and broccolini (or broccoli rabe) to the boiling water and cook until just tender, 3 to 5 minutes. Reserve 1 cup of the cooking water. Drain and transfer the pasta and vegetables to the skillet; toss to combine, adding enough of the reserved water to achieve desired consistency. Toss with parsley and salt and serve topped with almonds and goat cheese. Garnish with lemon zest, if desired.

30. Cheesy Ground Beef & Broccoli Casserole

Prep Time: 30 mins

Total Time: 30 mins

Servings: 4

Ingredients

- 1 pound 90%-lean ground beef
- 1 small yellow onion, finely chopped
- 4 cups chopped broccoli
- 3 tablespoons all-purpose flour
- 1 tablespoon chopped fresh sage
- 2 cloves garlic, finely chopped
- 1 ½ cups nonfat milk
- 4 ounces 1/3-less-fat cream cheese
- 1 cup shredded Cheddar cheese
- ½ teaspoon salt
- ¼ teaspoon ground pepper
- ⅔ cup panko breadcrumbs, preferably whole-wheat
- 1 tablespoon extra-virgin olive oil
- ½ teaspoon paprika

Directions

1. Position rack in upper third of oven; preheat broiler. Cook ground beef and onion in a large ovenproof nonstick skillet over medium heat, breaking the beef into bite-size pieces with a wooden spoon, until the beef is no longer pink, about 10 minutes. Add broccoli; cook, stirring occasionally, until the broccoli is tender-crisp, about 3 minutes. Add flour, sage and garlic; cook, stirring constantly, until the beef and vegetables are well coated in the flour mixture, about 1 minute.
2. Add milk and bring to a simmer over medium-high heat. Cook, stirring occasionally, until thickened, 1 to 2 minutes. Stir in cream cheese and Cheddar until melted, about 1 minute. Remove from heat and stir in salt and pepper.
3. Mix breadcrumbs, oil and paprika in a small bowl. Sprinkle evenly over the mixture in the skillet.
4. Broil the casserole until the breadcrumbs are golden brown and the edges are bubbling, 1 to 3 minutes.